Amene FKI
Mounira HAJJAJI
Walid FEKI

Determinants of smoking behaviour in a working population

Amene FKI
Mounira HAJJAJI
Walid FEKI

Determinants of smoking behaviour in a working population

ScienciaScripts

Imprint

Any brand names and product names mentioned in this book are subject to trademark, brand or patent protection and are trademarks or registered trademarks of their respective holders. The use of brand names, product names, common names, trade names, product descriptions etc. even without a particular marking in this work is in no way to be construed to mean that such names may be regarded as unrestricted in respect of trademark and brand protection legislation and could thus be used by anyone.

Cover image: www.ingimage.com

This book is a translation from the original published under ISBN 978-620-6-71183-4.

Publisher:
Sciencia Scripts
is a trademark of
Dodo Books Indian Ocean Ltd. and OmniScriptum S.R.L publishing group

120 High Road, East Finchley, London, N2 9ED, United Kingdom
Str. Armeneasca 28/1, office 1, Chisinau MD-2012, Republic of Moldova, Europe
Printed at: see last page
ISBN: 978-620-7-62204-7

PLAN

INTRODUCTION 2

MATERIALS AND METHODS 4

RESULTS 9

DISCUSSION 20

CONCLUSION 27

REFERENCES 30

APPENDICES 36

INTRODUCTION

Tobacco is one of the main causes of death in the world, but also the main preventable cause of death. It is responsible for nearly 6 million deaths a year worldwide and causes hundreds of billions of dollars in economic losses every year. Most of these deaths occur in low- and middle-income countries, and this gap is set to widen over the coming decades (1).

In Tunisia, the prevalence of smoking is still high, and it is expected that the consequences of smoking, in terms of mortality, will be even more serious in the next two decades, if effective anti-smoking measures are not put in place, in particular legislative and regulatory measures, effective educational measures and measures to help people stop smoking (2).

The relationship between smoking and work is still a hot topic. It is well documented that smoking seriously damages health and predicts occupational consequences such as disability (3), early retirement (4) and sickness absence (5). Currently, in developed countries, smoking in the workplace is almost completely banned or, at least, there are policies in place to tackle smoking, often combined with smoking cessation programmes. However, smoking remains a major problem for the majority of the world's working population, including Tunisia. And so it is always important to identify the factors linked to the working environment and work organisation that can contribute - positively or negatively - to determining smoking behaviour.

The hypothesis that the work environment could influence smoking behaviour is suggested on the basis of the following findings: the work environment can influence the probability of quitting smoking, the probability of relapse after initial cessation and the quantity of cigarettes smoked (1-3). These three relationships may not necessarily operate independently of each other. of the others, and different mechanisms could contribute to each of them. Firstly, stress factors at work could increase smoking or make it more difficult to stop (6-9). Secondly, resources in the work environment, such as decision latitude or rewards, could reinforce individual resources and thus make it possible to reduce smoking, stop smoking or avoid relapses (10). Thirdly, an imbalance between effort and reward may contribute to an increase in the frequency of smoking and difficulties in quitting (11).

Scientific studies on smoking in relation to work have produced conflicting results. Some authors have suggested that the work environment, impaired quality of life and high psychological demands at work play a well-established role in smoking behaviour (12,13). However, in other studies, stress at work was not strongly associated with heavy smoking (14,15).

As for smoking cessation, while for some authors it may be less likely in workplaces with high psychological stress and low control (16). For others, the importance of psychosocial factors at work was not a predictive factor for smoking cessation failure (17,18).

Given all these contradictory results and the absence of a formal link between stress experienced at work and smoking behaviour, the question arises as to the association between an effort/reward imbalance at work and smoking habits. This finding prompted us to study this association, particularly in a population of employees in a district of the national water exploitation and distribution company (SONEDE):

■Determine the prevalence of smoking in the population studied

■Assessing stress in the workplace
■Determine the factors influencing smoking behaviour, the level of dependence and motivation to stop smoking.

MATERIALS AND METHODS

1. Type of study :

The present study is a descriptive and analytical cross-sectional survey that took place in a district of the national water exploitation and distribution company (SONEDE) in Sfax and carried out over a period of 2 months (from 01 December 2017 to 31 January 2018).

2. Study population :

The study population consisted of male workers employed at SONEDE in Sfax, whether or not they were smokers. They were divided into 2 groups according to their type of activity:

► Active workers: are those whose activity is manual (mechanics, plumbers, electricians warehousemen, agents multi-skilled workers, drivers, security guards).

► Sedentary workers: are those whose activity is office-based (administrative staff, engineers, technicians, accountants).

Thepopulation was divided also into 2 groups according to smoking behaviour:

► Current non-smokers: never smokers and ex-smokers

► Current smokers

Before the start of the survey, and during a personal interview, each subject was informed of the objectives and practical conduct of the study, as well as their right to refuse to take part and/or to withdraw without having to provide any justification.

3. Data collection and variable definition :

Data were collected using a questionnaire comprising :

3.1. Demographic and socio-professional characteristics

The questionnaire enabled us to collect descriptive variables relating to the main socio-demographic characteristics, in particular age, level of education (primary, secondary or university), marital status (single, married, divorced or widowed), occupation and work organisation (nature of tasks, length of service, number of hours worked per week and overtime (yes/no)).

3.2. History of active smoking :

One section of the questionnaire was specific to smokers and concerned the history of active smoking (type of tobacco (cigarette, chicha and/or neffa), age of start-up, etc.), the average number of cigarettes smoked per day with the determination of three classes of consumption (low consumption (<10cigarettes/day), moderate consumption (between 11-20 cigarettes/day) and heavy consumption (>20cigarettes/day)), previous attempts to give up smoking (yes/no), the quantity in pack-years (PA) and other addictive behaviours (alcohol, coffee).

The level of tobacco dependence was assessed by the fagerström test:

• 0 to 2 points: no nicotine dependence

• 3 to 4 points: low nicotine dependence

• 5 to 6 points: moderate nicotine dependence

• 7 to 8 points: high nicotine dependence

• 9 to 10 points: very strong nicotine dependence

Motivation to quit smoking was assessed using the Largue and Légeron test:

- < 6: insufficient motivation

- 7 to 13: average motivation

- >13: good motivation

3-3- Measuring stress at work

The model used to characterise stress factors at work is Siegrist's Effort/Reward Imbalance model (19), which focuses on a negative trade-off between "Costs" and "Rewards" at work. In this model, a high workload is assumed to be an important extrinsic factor contributing to high effort expenditure. Low rewards, the other component of imbalance, refer to scarcity in terms of money, self-esteem and control of professional status.

The Siegrist questionnaire has 3 dimensions:

❖**Effort: score ranging from 6 to 30**

Score = item1 + item2 + item3 + item4 + item5 + item6

❖**Rewards: scores ranging from 11 to 55**

Score = item7 + item8 + item9 + item10 + item11 + item12 + item13 + item14 + item15 + item16 + item17

❖**Over-investment: score ranging from 6 to 24**

Score = item18 + item19 + (5 - item20) + item21 + item22 + item23

The over-investment score is then dichotomised at the upper tertile of the distribution in the study sample, i.e. a threshold of 18 in our sample:

- <18: no over-investment
- ≥18: presence of overinvestment

❖**Building the effort/reward ratio**

Ratio= 11/6 x effort score / (66 - reward score)

A ratio > 1 defines employees exposed to an imbalance between effort and reward.

4. Statistical tools :

The data collected was entered and processed using SPSS20 software.

4.1. Descriptive study

In the descriptive section, we listed all the characteristics of the population studied. Qualitative variables were presented in the form of frequencies and percentages. Quantitative variables were expressed as averages.

4.2. Analytical study

In the univariate study, percentages were compared using the Chi 2 test or the Fisher exact test, and means were compared using Student's t-test. The significance level was set at 5%, and differences were considered significant if $p<0.05$.

For the level of smoking dependence, we defined 2 groups:

• No dependency: includes non-dependent smokers and low-dependency smokers.

• Dependence: includes moderately dependent smokers and those who are heavily to very heavily dependent.

For motivation to stop smoking, we also defined 2 groups:

• Unmotivated: for smokers with insufficient motivation.

• Motivated: grouping together smokers with average and good motivation.

We completed a multivariate analysis using binary logistic regression to identify the factors influencing smoking behaviour, nicotine dependence and motivation to stop smoking.

5. Bibliographic research

The bibliographic search was carried out using the following search engines: "science direct.com", "em-consulte.com" and "pubmed.com", using the following keywords: smoking, workers, stress,

6. Ethical considerations

Patient anonymity was respected. The study was conducted with strict respect for medical confidentiality with no conflict of interest.

RESULTS

1. Socio-demographic characteristics of the population studied

Seventy-one male employees took part in the survey, representing a participation rate of 67.61% (71/105).

1.1. Age

The average age of employees was 43.96 +/- 11.06 years, with extremes ranging from 23 to 59 years.

1.2. Marital status

The majority of employees (78.9%) were married (Figure 1).

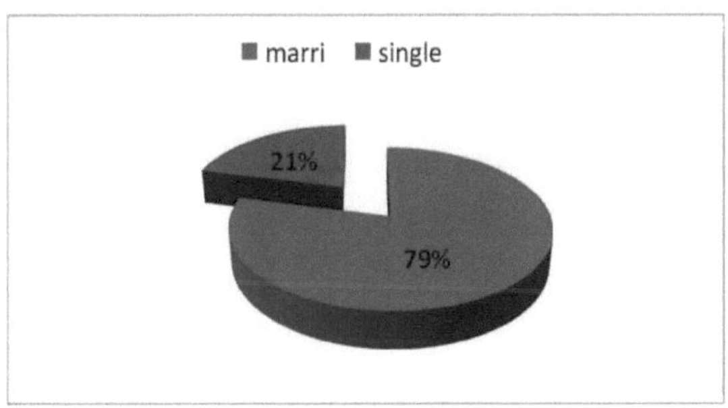

Figure 1: Breakdown of the population by marital status

1.3. Level of study

More than half the employees (57.7%) had a secondary education (table I).

Table I: Breakdown of the population by level of education

Level of study	Workforce	Percentage
Primary	14	19,7
Secondary	41	57,7
University	16	22,6
Total	71	100

2. Professional features

2.1. Type of activity

More than half of all employees (56%) were in work (Figure 2).

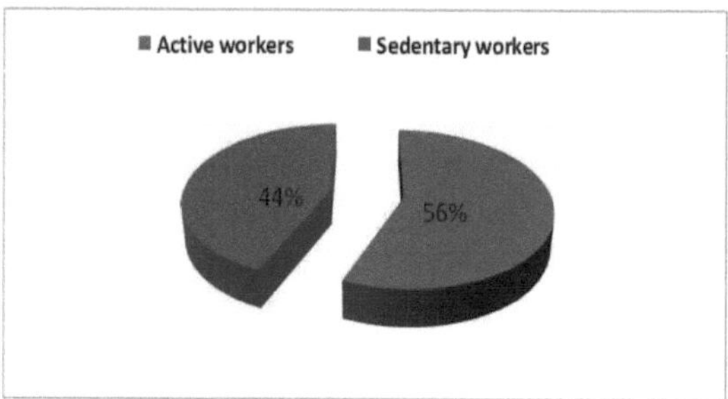

Figure 2: Breakdown of employees by type of activity

2.2. Workstation

The majority of sedentary employees were administrative staff (18.3%) and engineers (11.3%). The majority of active employees were mechanics (12.7%) and multi-skilled workers (8.5%) (Table II).

Table II: Breakdown of employees by workstation
Sedentary workers

Profession	Workforce	Percentage
Administrative agents	13	18,3
	8	11,3
	4	5,6
Technicians	5	7
Accountants	3	4,2
Mechanics	9	12,7
Storekeepers	6	8,5
Lifters	6	8,5
Plumbers	5	7
Active workers Turners	2	2,8
Drivers	2	2,8
Electrician	1	1,4
Security agent	1	1,4
Multi-skilled workers	6	8,5
Total	71	100

Section Head Engineers

2.3. Length of service

The average length of service was 18.5 years +/- 11.6 years, with extremes ranging from 1 year to 38 years.

2.4. Pace of work

The average number of hours worked per week was 40.8 +/- 2.08 hours. Almost one quarter of employees (22,5%) performed overtime overtime.

3. Study of smoking behaviour

3.1. Prevalence of smoking in the study population

Sixty-two per cent of employees used to smoke and 13% have stopped (Figure 3).

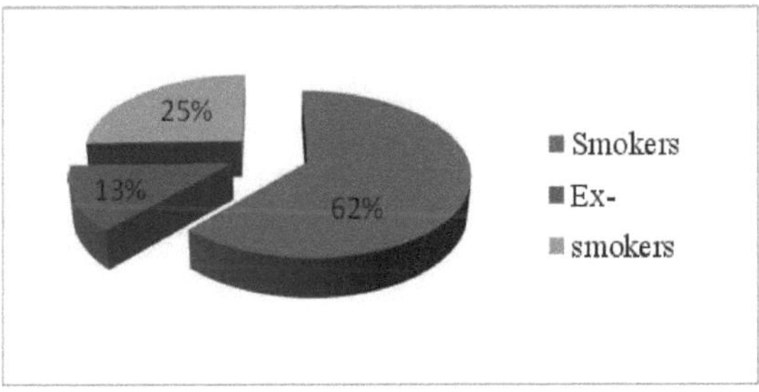

Figure 3: Breakdown of employees by smoking profile

3.2. Age of onset of smoking

The average age of smoking initiation was 17.7 ± 3.5 years, with extremes ranging from 8 to 26 years.

3.3. uantity of smoking

The average number of cigarettes smoked per day was 19.5, ranging from 5 to 40 cigarettes. The majority (74.6%) smoked moderately (between 11 and 20 cigarettes a day) (Figure 4).

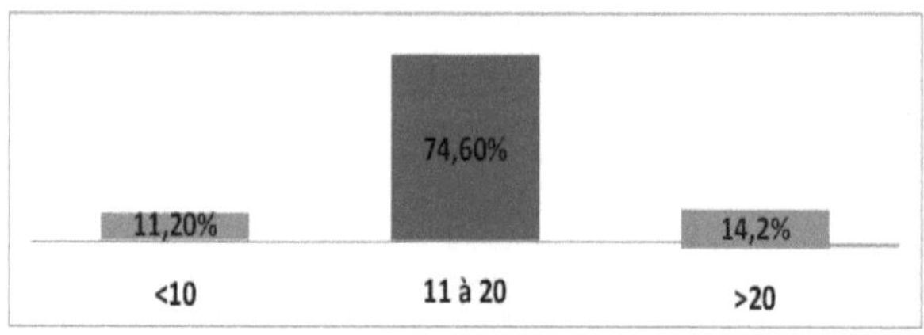

Figure 4: Breakdown of smokers by number of cigarettes smoked per day

The average number of year packs (YP) was 22.5 and ranged from 5 to 63 YP.

3.4.Smoking in the workplace

All the employees who smoked said they had smoked at work, 93% of them outside their breaks.

3.5.Assessing smokers' knowledge of the harmful effects of tobacco

All employees who smoked said they were aware of the harmful effects of tobacco on health, but only 22.7% had received education on how to stop smoking.

3.6.Attempts to stop smoking

Most smokers (84.1%) had tried to quit one or more times, with an average of two attempts.

3.7.Assessment of nicotine dependence

According to the Fagerstrom questionnaire, 31.8% of smokers were highly dependent on tobacco (table III).

Table III: Breakdown of smokers by level of dependence on tobacco

Level of dependence	Workforce	Percentage
Absent (0 to 2)	10	22,7
Low (3 to 4)	9	20,5
Average (5 to 6)	10	22,7
Strong (7 to 8)	14	31,8
Very strong (9 to 10)	1	2,3
Total	44	100

3.8. Assessing motivation to stop smoking

According to the Largue and Légeron test, 40.9% of smoking employees were insufficiently motivated to stop smoking (table IV).

Table IV: Breakdown of smokers by level of motivation to stop smoking

Level of motivation	Workforce	Percentage
Insufficient (score < 6)	18	40,9
Average (score 7 to 13)	15	34,1
Good (score > 13)	11	25
Total	44	100

3.9. Other adductive pipes

3.9.1. Alcoholism

The majority of employees were non-alcoholic in 87.3% of cases.

3.9.2. Café

The majority of employees (94.4%) drank coffee, with an average of 2 cups per day. Smokers consumed more coffee than non-smokers, with a statistically significant difference (p= 0.020).

4. Effort/reward imbalance

According to the Siegrist model, 35.2% of employees had an imbalance between effort and reward at work (ratio > 1) (Table V).

Table V: Distribution according to the presence or absence of an effort-reward imbalance

Imbalance

effort/reward	Workforce	Percentage
Yes	25	35,2
No	46	64,8

5. Over-investment at work

The presence of over-investment in work concerned 33.8% of the employees (table VI).

Table VI: Distribution according to the presence or absence of over-investment in work

Overinvestment	Workforce	Percentage
Yes	24	33,8
No	47	66,2

6. Determinants of smoking behaviour

6.1. Univariate analysis

Active workers were at greater risk of smoking than sedentary workers (p=0.038; OR=2.80; 95% CI [1.04 - 7.57]). An effort/reward imbalance was more frequent in current smokers than in current non-smokers, with a statistically significant difference (p= 0.021; OR= 3.66; 95% CI [1.17 - 11.44]) (table VII).

Table VII: Determinants of smoking behaviour in the univariate analysis

Socio-professional factors

Current smokers Number (%) current

Non-smokers Type de Number of smokers (%)	P ORIC 95% confidence interval		
43,96 ± 11,8 Student	0,99	-	-
4 (26,7)Chi-square	0,3	-	-
4 (28,6) 17 (41,5) Chi-square 6 (37,5)	0,69	-	-
11 (27,5)Khi-deux	0,03	2,8	[1,04 - 7,57]
18,81 ± 12Student	0,87	-	-
41,2 ± 2,8Student	0,21	-	-
4 (25)Chi-square	0,22	-	-
5 (20)Chi-square	0,02	3,6	[1,17 - 11,4]
8 (33,3)Chi-square	0,56	-	-

test

Age (mean) 43.95 ± 11.12

Marital status Single	11 (73,3)	
Married	33 (58,9)	23 (41,1)
Primary	10 (71,4)	
Level of study Secondary	24 (58,5)	
University	10 (62,5)	
Type of activity Active	29 (72,5)	
Sedentary	15 (48,4)	16 (51,6)
Seniority	18,36 ± 11,3	
Number of hours/week	40,52 ± 1,4	
Overtime Oui	12 (75)	
No	32 (58,2)	23 (41,8)
Imbalance Yes	20 (80)	
effort/reward No	24 (52,2)	22 (47,8)
Overinvestment Oui	16 (66,7)	
No	28 (59,6)	19 (40,4)

6.2. Multivariate analysis

In the multivariate analysis, smoking status was associated only with the type of activity (p=0.044; OR = 0.205; 95% CI [0.044 - 0.962]) (table VIII).

Table VIII: Determinants of smoking behaviour in the multivariate analysis

95% CI for OR

Smoking behaviour	p	OR	Lower	Superior
Age	0,465	-	-	-
Family situation	0,194	-	-	-
Level of study	0,267	-	-	-
Length of service	0,785	-	-	-
Type of activity	0,044	0,205	,044	,962
Effort-reward imbalance	0,425	-	-	-
Overinvestment	0,845	-	-	-

7. Factors determining the level of dependence on tobacco

7.1. Univariate analysis

Nicotine dependence was statistically associated with sedentary activity (p= 0.03; OR= 4.4; 95% CI [1.17 - 16.9]) and an imbalance between effort and reward (p= 0.001; OR = 11.3; 95% CI [2.5 - 50.3]) (table IX).

Table IX: Determinants of tobacco dependence in univariate analysis

Facteurs socioprofessionnels		Dépendance		Type de test	p	OR	IC à 95%
		Non Effectif (%)	Oui Effectif (%)				
Age (moyenne)		$44 \pm 11,1$	$43,9 \pm 11,3$	Student	0,9	-	-
Situation matrimoniale	Célibataire	5 (45,5)	6 (54,5)	Ficher	1	-	-
	Marié	14 (42,4)	19 (57,6)				
Niveau d'étude	Primaire	2 (20)	8 (80)	Ficher	0,23	-	-
	Secondaire	11 (50)	11 (50)				
	Universitaire	6 (50)	6 (50)				
Type d'activité	Active	9 (31)	20 (69)	Khi-deux	0,03	4,4	[1,1-16,9]
	Sédentaire	10 (66,7)	5 (33,3)				
Ancienneté professionnelle		$19,8 \pm 12,5$	$17,2 \pm 10,5$	Student	0,44	-	-
Nombre heures/semaine		$40,3 \pm 1,1$	$40,6 \pm 1,6$	Student	0,4	-	-
Heures supplémentaires	Oui	4 (33,3)	8 (66,7)	Khi-deux	0,5	-	-
	Non	15 (46,9)	17 (53,1)				
Déséquilibre efforts/ récompenses	Oui	3 (15)	17 (85)	Khi-deux	0,001	11,3	[2,5-50,3]
	Non	16 (66,7)	8 (33,3)				
Surinvestissement	Oui	6 (37,5)	10 (62,5)	Khi-deux	0,56	-	-
	Non	10 (46,4)	15 (53,6)				

7.2. Multivariate analysis

In the multivariate analysis, smoking dependence was associated with the presence of an effort/reward imbalance (p=0.029; OR = 10.06; 95% CI [1.26 - 80.45]) (Table X).

Table X: Determinants of tobacco dependence in the multivariate analysis

Tobacco dependence	p	OR	95% CI for OR	
			Lower	Higher
Age	0,659	-	-	-
Family situation	0,641	-	-	-
Level of study	0,985	-	-	-
Length of service	0,367	-	-	-
Type of activity	0,388	-	-	-
Overtime	0,525	-	-	-
Effort/reward imbalance	0,029	10,068	1,260	80,457
Overinvestment	0,369	-	-	-

8. Determinants of motivation to stop smoking

8.1. Univariate analysis

Motivation to stop smoking was associated with sedentary activity (p=0.04; OR= 0.23; 95% CI [0.05-0.9]) (table XI).

Table XI: Determinants of motivation to quit smoking in the univariate analysis

Facteurs Socioprofessionnels		Motivation		Type de Test	p	OR	IC à 95%
		Oui Effectif (%)	Non Effectif (%)				
Age (moyenne)		41,8 ± 11	46,9 ±10,9	Student	0,14	-	-
Situation Matrimoniale	Célibataire	7 (63,6)	4 (36,4)	Fisher	1	-	-
	Marié	19 (57,6)	14 (42,4)				
Niveau d'étude	Primaire	4 (40)	6 (60)	Fisher	0,24	-	-
	Secondaire	13 (59,1)	9 (40,9)				
	Universitaire	9 (75)	3 (25)				
Type d'activité	Active	14 (48,3)	15 (51,7)	Khi-deux	0,04	0,2	0,05-0, 9
	Sédentaire	12 (80)	3 (20)				
Ancienneté professionnelle (moyenne)		15,9 ± 11,1	21,8 ± 10,9	Student	0,08	-	-
Heures supplémentaires	Oui	5 (41,7)	7 (58,3)	Fisher	0,18	-	-
	Non	21 (65,6)	11 (34,4)				
Déséquilibre efforts/ récompenses	Oui	11 (55)	9 (45)	Khi-deux	0,61	-	-
	Non	15 (62,5)	9 (37,5)				
Surinvestissement	Oui	10 (62,5)	6 (37,5)	Khi-deux	0,72	-	-
	Non	16 (57,1)	12 (42,9)				

8.2. Multivariate analysis

In the multivariate analysis, motivation to stop smoking was associated with sedentary-type activity (p = 0.03; OR = 27.65; 95% CI [1.38 - 552.3]) (table XII).

Table XII: Determinants of motivation to stop smoking in the analysis

Multivariate

	95% OR Motivation to quit	p	OR	Lower	Higher
Age		0,731	-	-	-
Family situation		0,083	-	-	-
Level of study		0,317	-	-	-
Length of service		0,100	-	-	-
Sedentary activity		0,030	27,650	1,384	552,340
Overtime		0,547	-	-	-
Effort/reward imbalance		0,781	-	-	-
Overinvestment		0,795	-	-	-

DISCUSSION

The issue of smoking in the workplace remains a topical one. The absence of a formal link between the psychosocial risks experienced at work and smoking behaviour underlines the importance of studying the effects of these risks on smoking behaviour, tobacco dependency and low motivation to quit among a population of employees of a water exploitation and distribution company.

1. Strengths and weaknesses of the study

Our study has a number of strong points that deserve to be highlighted mentioned :

▶ The survey is relatively easy to carry out.

▶ Its duration is short.

▶ It is reproducible and relatively inexpensive.

▶ Use of standardised and validated questionnaires to assess smoking dependency, motivation to stop smoking and the effort/reward imbalance, thereby reducing measurement bias.

▶ Taking into account certain non-work-related factors, analysing and evaluation of confounding variables.

Despite the strengths of our study, certain limitations should be mentioned:

▶ Bias due to the non-response of certain workers (participation rate = 67.6%)

▶ Small sample size, which poses a problem in terms of power test statistics.

▶ Type of study: cross-sectional study, therefore we do not claim that the associations observed are proof of a true relationship. longitudinal studies are needed to confirm these associations.

▶ This study concerns employees of a specific company, which means that may make it difficult to extrapolate these results to the general population.

► Self-declaration of workers in response to the questionnaire questionnaire at Effort/reward imbalance may be a source of bias due to individual differences in the perception, experience and interpretation of psychosocial factors at work. An alternative approach could be to model the effect of ERI (effort/reward imbalance) with the addition of a score at the level of each work unit - for example, by assigning an aggregate mean ERI score in each work unit to each participant, this would allow a multi-level analytical approach to be used (20).

2. Prevalence of smoking

The prevalence of smoking in our study population was estimated at 63%. This prevalence is higher than that estimated by Fakhfakh R et al.(2) among manual workers, service personnel, employees and middle managers (48.3% to 54.4%). It is also much higher than that reported in a meta-analysis of 15 European studies involving 166,130 workers (smoking prevalence was 25%) (21) and also in another study conducted in 10 municipalities and 21 hospitals in Finland, where smoking prevalence among male workers was estimated at 25% (22).

3. Determinants of smoking behaviour

3.1. Type of activity :

In our study, smoking was more prevalent among active workers than sedentary workers (p=0.038; OR=2.80; 95% CI [1.04 - 7.57]). This result was consistent with several studies in the literature, such as a study of male Kôrin workers (23), in which the prevalence of smoking was higher in active workers than in office workers (OR= 2.00, 95% CI [1.43 - 2.80]; PR= 1.33, CI 95% [1.12 - 1.59]), this difference increased from 1998 to 2005, then decreased from 2005 to 2009. Overall, these results indicate that the difference in smoking rates between these two occupational categories has decreased since 2005, although smoking remains more likely and more prevalent among active workers. Other epidemiological studies have also shown that smoking behaviour varies between socio-economic classes (24,25) and between different job categories (26,27), with a higher proportion of smokers and heavy smokers in the lowest socio-economic classes and in "blue collar" occupations. Differences in smoking rates of 20-30% between the lowest and highest socio-economic classes have been reported (25,28). The processes by which these social differences in smoking are formed and maintained are not well documented, but there are at least two plausible hypotheses: (1) that these differences are due to selection and (2) that they are due to the influence of social factors and the occupational environment. For the majority of smokers, smoking is a habit that is established before entering the labour market, which is in favour of the selection hypothesis. However, some studies have revealed large differences in smoking cessation rates between different jobs (29,30). In the United States in 1997, the prevalence of smoking among workers at "The proportion of blue-collar workers was almost twice that of white-collar workers (37% versus 21%). These disparities were also observed among female workers (33% among 'blue-collar' women vs. 20% among 'white-collar' workers). In addition, the smoking rate fell more slowly among active workers than among other workers (27). An analysis of data from the National Health Interview Survey (NHIS) in the United States in 2000 (31) revealed that smoking prevalence was higher among the most disadvantaged occupational categories, with low levels of education and low income, and that each of these indicators of socio-economic development was positively associated with smoking prevalence. These disparities reflect wider structural problems involving a range of socio-economic factors that ultimately have significant effects on health and adductive behaviour (32).For example, the results of the Alameda County study showed that behaviours such as smoking are associated with low income and vary according to socio-economic background (33). Similarly, Graham (34) reported that social contextual factors associated with low income are particularly related to smoking habits.All these findings on smoking prevalence by occupational category highlight the need for new approaches to tobacco control in the workplace.

3.2. Effort/reward imbalance

According to the Siegrist model, 35.2% of employees had an imbalance between effort and reward at work (ratio > 1). This imbalance was more frequent among current smokers than current non-smokers, with a statistically significant difference (p= 0.021; OR= 3.66 ; 95% CI [1.17 - 11.44]). This result was consistent with several studies reporting an association between effort/reward imbalance (35) and smoking. In a Finnish study of 46,190 workers, Kouvonen et al (22) reported that a high effort/reward ratio was associated with smoking (OR= 1.28). After taking into account age, level of education, professional status, type of employment and marital status, employees who had more stress at work were found to be smokers more often than their colleagues who had less stress. Similarly, in a cohort study conducted in the United States, psychosocial stress was associated with smoking behaviour in working adults (15).However, other studies have not reported an association between work stress and smoking (36-39). Indeed, a study in India (40) did not reveal a significant association between the different domains of the effort/reward imbalance score and the presence of adductive habits, but a significant association was found between a ratio ≥1 and smoking.

4. Factors determining the level of dependence on tobacco :

4.1. Type of activity :

Active workers had a higher level of nicotine dependence than sedentary workers (p= 0.03; OR= 4.4; 95% CI [1.17 - 16.9]). This result was consistent with the study conducted in Korai (23) on male workers in whom heavy smoking (>20 cigarettes/day) was more common among those performing manual activities. According to the authors, this difference between the two groups in terms of smoking intensity indicates that anti-smoking policies were less effective among active workers than sedentary workers. A low level of education was also reported as a factor linked to the quantity of cigarettes smoked (41). Other epidemiological studies have also shown that smoking dependence varies between different job categories (26,27,29), with a higher proportion of heavy smokers in "blue collar" occupations.

4.2. Effort/reward imbalance

The level of tobacco dependence was strongly associated with an imbalance between effort and reward (p= 0.001; OR = 11.3; 95% CI [2.5 - 50.3]). This result was consistent with the study by Kouvonen et al. (22) who showed that a high effort-reward ratio was associated with greater smoking intensity (OR= 1.19). Peter et al (42) also observed a positive association between the effort-reward ratio and smoking intensity in a cross-sectional study conducted in Germany. In the systematic review conducted by Albertsen et al (43), variations in the amount smoked among smokers were directly influenced by workplace demands. However, an Australian study (n= 1,101) found that a high effort-reward ratio was associated with greater tobacco dependence in women but not in men (44).Similarly, a study of office staff in India found no association between nicotine dependence and work-related stress (40).Potential mechanisms linking work stress to adductive behaviours are suggested on the basis of pathophysiological evidence. In terms of biological mechanisms, work stress can lead to biological responses (e.g. dysfunction of the meso-limbic /dopaminergic system in the brain), which result in dependence on a substance (alcohol or tobacco) (45). In terms of psychological mechanisms, stress at work predicts psychological distress such as anxiety and depression; these individuals will then adopt health-risk behaviours (focused on coping emotions) to temporarily relieve or avoid their psychological distress and distract their attention from the stressful situation (46).In our study, tobacco dependence was not associated with the presence of over-investment in work (p= 0.56), which is inconsistent with the literature. Indeed, Jenkins et al (47) reported that investment in work was present in 53% of heavy smokers (> 20 cigarettes per day), 47% of occasional smokers (< 20 cigarettes per day), and 41% of non-smokers. They then concluded that over-investment was associated with smoking status after 4 years of follow-up. Shekelle et al (48) also found that over-investment in work was positively associated with smoking intensity (number of cigarettes smoked per day) in a cross-sectional study of 4108 adults in the United States.

5. Professional factors determining motivation to stop smoking

In our study, motivation to quit smoking was associated only with the type of sedentary activity (p=0.04; OR= 0.23; 95% CI [0.05- 0.9]). In fact, 80% of sedentary workers were motivated to stop smoking, compared with 48.3% of active workers. This result was consistent with a number of studies that have found large differences in smoking cessation rates between different professions (29,30), which these authors believe may be influenced by the selection of higher educational levels and more personal resources for quitting smoking in socioeconomic classes. the highest. Low socio-economic status was also reported to be a factor in smoking cessation failure (49). In our study, motivation to stop smoking was not associated with the presence of an effort/reward imbalance. This same result was reported by Ota et al (50) who found that the effort-reward ratio was not a predictive factor for smoking cessation after 2 years of follow-up of 1423 adults in Japan.Similarly, in a meta-analysis of 15 European studies (18), significant associations between job strain and smoking cessation were not reported. Another Japanese study of male workers (17) found no link between high levels of job stress and low smoking cessation rates.However, other studies have reported a link between smoking cessation and stress at work. Indeed, Kouvonen (22) reported that smoking cessation was more frequent among employees with low work effort. Similarly, in the systematic review carried out in Europe (43), the probability of quitting smoking was higher among smokers with a higher level of resources at work and a sufficient level of demand, and relapse after quitting was more frequent the more stressful the demands became. In contrast, the Danish cohort study showed that smokers with high work demands were the most likely to stop smoking (51).

CONCLUSION

Smoking is a major risk factor for many diseases, and its impact on overall health is far from negligible. It is influenced by various characteristics of the population studied, in particular socio-professional category. To date, the determinants of smoking behaviour in relation to professional constraints are not well understood. Understanding the determinants of smoking behaviour is an important element in helping healthcare professionals to develop anti-smoking prevention initiatives and adopt strategies to help people stop smoking. In this context, we conducted a survey of a population of employees in a district of the national water exploitation and distribution company (SONEDE), the objectives of which were to determine the prevalence of smoking in the population studied, to evaluate work-related stress in this population and to determine the factors influencing smoking behaviour, the level of dependence on tobacco and motivation to stop smoking.The present study is a descriptive and analytical cross-sectional survey that took place in a district of the national water exploitation and distribution company (SONEDE) in Sfax and carried out over a period of 2 months (from 01 December 2017 to 31 January 2018). The study population consisted of male workers. They were divided according to their type of activity into 2 groups: active workers and sedentary workers with an office activity. The population was also divided into 2 groups according to their smoking behaviour: the group of current non-smokers and the group of current smokers. The data were collected using a questionnaire specifying demographic and socio-professional characteristics, in particular age, level of education, marital status, profession and work organisation. work. One section of the questionnaire was specific to smokers and concerned the history of smoking, the average number of cigarettes smoked per day, previous attempts to give up smoking, the number of cigarettes smoked in a packet per year (PA) and other addictive behaviours (alcohol, coffee). The level of smoking dependence was assessed by the Fagerstrom test, and motivation to stop smoking was assessed by the Largue and Légeron test. The model used to characterise stress factors at work is Siegrist's effort-reward imbalance model, which comprises 3 dimensions (effort, reward and over-investment) enabling a ratio to be calculated (a ratio > 1 defines employees exposed to an effort-reward imbalance).Seventy-one male employees took part in the survey, representing a participation rate of 67.61% (71/105). The average age of the employees was 43.96 +/- 11.06 years. The majority of employees (78.9%) were married. More than half of the employees (57.7%) had a secondary education. More than half of the employees (56%) were active workers. The majority of sedentary employees were administrative staff (18.3%) and engineers (11.3%). The majority of active employees were mechanics (12.7%) and multi-skilled workers (8.5%). The average length of service was 18.5 years +/- 11.6 years. The prevalence of smoking in the study population was 62%. The average age at which smoking began was 17.7 ± 3.5 years. The average number of cigarettes smoked per day was 19.5. The majority (74.6%) were moderate smokers. All the employees who smoked stated that they were aware of the harmful effects of tobacco on their health, but only 22.7% had received education on how to stop smoking.According to the Fagerstrom questionnaire, 31.8% of smokers were highly dependent on tobacco, and according to the Largue and Légeron test, 40.9% were insufficiently motivated to stop smoking. Regarding the evaluation of stress at work, according to the Siegrist model, 35.2% of employees had a /-+. effort-reward imbalance (ratio > 1) and 33.8% were over-invested in their work. In the univariate analysis, active workers were more at risk of being smokers than sedentary workers (p=0.038; OR=2.80; 95% CI [1.04 - 7.57]), more dependent on tobacco (p= 0.03; OR= 4.4; 95% CI [1.17 - 16.9]), and had lower motivation to stop smoking (p=0.04; OR= 0.23; 95% CI [0.05-0.9]). The presence of an effort-reward imbalance was associated with smoking behaviour (p= 0.021; OR= 3.66; 95% CI [1.17 - 11.44]) and smoking dependence (p= 0.001; OR = 11.3; 95% CI [2.5 - 50.3]).In the multivariate analysis, manual-type activity was associated with smoking status (p=0.044; OR = 0.205; 95% CI [0.044 - 0.962]) and motivation to stop smoking (p=0.03; OR = 27.65; 95% CI [1.38 - 552.3]), while smoking dependence was associated with the presence of an effort-reward imbalance (p=0.029; OR = 10.06; 95% CI [1.26 - 80.45]).Our results suggest that reducing stress at work by ensuring a better balance between personal effort and the rewards obtained could prevent smoking. Studies of smoking cessation interventions combined with stress management interventions would therefore be an important step in promoting employee health.

REFERENCES

1. World Health Organization. Report on the global tobacco epidemic 2011. Warning About Dangers Tab.

2. Fakhfakh R, Hsairi M, Achour N. [Epidemiology and prevention of smoking in Tunisia : current situation and perspectives] Epidemiology and prevention of tobacco use in Tunisia : a review. 2001;(January 2014).

3. Krokstad, S., Johnsen, R., Westin S. Social determinants of disability pension: a 10-year follow-up of 62,000 people in a Norwegian county population. Int J Epidemiol. 2002;31(6):1183-91.

4. Lund T, Iversen L, Poulsen KB. Work environment factors, health, lifestyle and marital status as predictors of job change and early retirement in physically heavy occupations. Am J Ind Med. 2001 Aug;40(2):161-9.

5. Wooden M, Bush R. Smoking cessation and absence from work. Prev Med (Baltim). 1995 Sep;24(5):535-40.

6. Cohen S, Lichtenstein E. Perceived stress, quitting smoking, and smoking relapse. Heal Psychol. 1990;9(4):466-78.

7. Serxner S, Catalano R, Dooley D, Mishra S. Tobacco use: selection, stress, or culture? J Occup Med. 1991 Oct;33(10):1035-9.

8. Steptoe A, Wardle J, Pollard TM, Canaan L, Davies GJ. Stress, social support and health-related behavior: a study of smoking, alcohol consumption and physical exercise. J Psychosom Res. 1996 Aug;41(2):171-80.

9. Westman M, Eden D, Shirom A. Job stress, cigarette smoking and cessation: The conditioning effects of peer support. Soc Sci Med. Pergamon; 1985 Jan 1;20(6):637-44.

10. Pucci, L.G., Haglund B. Organizational factors affecting smoking at work: results from focus group interviews with smokers and ex-smokers. J Prim Prev. 1993;14(2):115-27.

11. Cohen S, Schwartz JE, Bromet EJ, Parkinson DK. Mental health, stress, and poor health behaviors in two community samples. Prev Med (Baltim). 1991 Mar;20(2):306-15.

12. Brisson C, Larocque B, Moisan J, Vézina M, Dagenais GR. Psychosocial factors at work, smoking, sedentary behavior, and body mass index: a prevalence study among 6995 white collar workers. J Occup Environ Med. 2000 Jan;42(1):40-6.

13. Tsutsumi A, Kayaba K, Yoshimura M, Sawada M, Ishikawa S, Sakai K, et al. Association between job characteristics and health behaviors in Japanese rural workers. Int J Behav Med. 2003;10(2):125-42.

14. Kouvonen A, Vahtera J, Väänänen A, Vogli R De, Heponiemi T, Elovainio M, et al. Relationship between job strain and smoking cessation: the Finnish Public Sector Study. Tob Control. 2009 Apr;18(2):108-14.
15. Slopen N, Zobel Kontos E, Ryff CD, Ayanian JZ, Albert MA, Williams DR. Psychosocial stress and cigarette smoking persistence, cessation, and relapse over 9-10 years: A prospective study of middle-aged adults in the United States NIH Public Access. Cancer Causes Control. 2013;24(10):1849-63.

16. Ota A, Masue T, Yasuda N, Tsutsumi A, Mino Y, Ohara H, et al. Psychosocial job characteristics and smoking cessation: A prospective cohort study using the Demand- Control-Support and Effort-Reward Imbalance job stress models. Nicotine Tob Res. 2010 Mar;12(3):287-93.

17. Fukuoka E, Hirokawa K, Kawakami N, Tsuchiya M, Haratani T, Kobayashi F, et al. Job strain and smoking cessation among Japanese male employees: a two-year follow-up study. Acta Med Okayama. 2008 Apr;62(2):83-91.

18. Heikkilä K, Nyberg ST, Fransson EI, Alfredsson L, De Bacquer D, Bjorner JB, et al. Job strain and tobacco smoking: an individual-participant data meta-analysis of 166,130 adults in 15 European studies. Mazza M, editor. PLoS One. 2012 Jul 6;7(7):e35463.

19. Siegrist J. Adverse health effects of high-effort/low-reward conditions. J Occup Health Psychol. 1996 Jan;1(1):27-41.

20. Elovainio M, Pentti J, Linna A, Virtanen M, Vahtera J. Observational study in a large occupational cohort. 2006;422-7.

21. Nyberg ST, Fransson EI, Alfredsson L, Bacquer D De, Bjorner JB, Hamer M, et al. Job Strain and Tobacco Smoking: An Individual- Participant Data Meta-Analysis of 166 130 Adults in 15 European Studies. 2012;7(7).

22. Kouvonen A, Kivima M, Virtanen M, Pentti J, Vahtera J. Work stress, smoking status, and smoking intensity: an observational study of 46 190 employees. 2005;63-9.

23. Kim BG, Pang DD, Park YJ, Lee JI, Kim HR, Myong JP, et al. Heavy smoking rate trends and related factors in Korean occupational groups: analysis of KNHANES 2007- 2012 data. BMJ Open. 2015;5(11):e008229.

24. Borg V, Kristensen TS. Social class and self-rated health: can the gradient be explained by differences in life style or work environment? Soc Sci Med. Pergamon; 2000 Oct 1;51(7):1019-30.

25. Marmot MG, Smith GD, Stansfeld S, Patel C, North F, Head J, et al. Health inequalities among British civil servants: the Whitehall II study. Lancet (London, England). Elsevier; 1991 Jun 8;337(8754):1387-93.

26. Leigh JP. Occupations, cigarette smoking, and lung cancer in the epidemiological follow-up to the NHANES I and the California Occupational Mortality Study. Bull N Y Acad Med. 1996;73(2):370-97.

27. Nelson DE, Emont SL, Brackbill RM, Cameron LL, Peddicord J, Fiore MC. Cigarette smoking prevalence by occupation in the United States. A comparison between 1978 to 1980 and 1987 to 1990. J Occup Med. 1994 May;36(5):516-25.

28. Osler M, Gerdes LU, Davidsen M, Brønnum-Hansen H, Madsen M, Jørgensen T, et al. Socioeconomic status and trends in risk factors for cardiovascular diseases in the Danish MONICA population, 1982-1992. J Epidemiol Community Health. BMJ Publishing Group; 2000 Feb;54(2):108-13.

29. Lundberg O, Rosén B, Rosén M. Who stopped smoking? Results from a panel survey of living conditions in Sweden. Soc Sci Med. 1991;32(5):619-22.

30. Osler M. Social class and health behaviour in Danish adults: a longitudinal study. Public Health. 1993 Jul;107(4):251-60.

31. Barbeau EM, Krieger N, Soobader M-J. Working class matters: socioeconomic disadvantage, race/ethnicity, gender, and smoking in NHIS 2000. Am J Public Health. American Public Health Association; 2004 Feb;94(2):269-78.

32. Freudenberg N. Time for a national agenda to improve the health of urban populations. Am J Public Health. American Public Health Association; 2000 Jun;90(6):837-40.

33. GA K. Where do shared pathways lead? Some reflections on a research agenda. Psychosom Med. 1995;57:208-2012.

34. Graham H. Promoting health against inequality: using research to identify targets for intervention - a case study of women and smoking. Health Educ J. Sage PublicationsSage CA: Thousand Oaks, CA; 1998 Dec 24;57(4):292-302.

35. Peter R. . Job stressors, coping characteristics, and the development of coronary heart disease (CHD): results from two studies. PsychologischeBeitrage. 1995;37:40-5.

36. Landsbergis PA, Schnall PL, Deitz DK, Warren K, Pickering TG, Schwartz JE. Job strain and health behaviors: results of a prospective study. Am J Health Promot. 1998 Mar 26;12(4):237-45.

37. Reed DM, LaCroix AZ, Karasek RA, Miller D, MacLean CA. Occupational strain and the incidence of coronary heart disease. Am J Epidemiol. 1989 Mar;129(3):495-502.

38. van Loon AJ, Tijhuis M, Surtees PG, Ormel J. Lifestyle risk factors for cancer: the relationship with psychosocial work environment. Int J Epidemiol. 2000 Oct;29(5):785- 92.

39. Netterstrøm B, Kristensen TS, Damsgaard MT, Olsen O, Sjøl A. Job strain and cardiovascular risk factors: a cross sectional study of employed Danish men and women. Br J Ind Med. 1991 Oct;48(10):684-9.

40. Priyanka R, Rao A, Rajesh G, Shenoy R. Work-Associated Stress and Nicotine Dependence among Law Enforcement Personnel in Mangalore , India. 2016;17:829-33.

41. Giskes K, Kunst AE, Benach J, Borrell C, Costa G, Dahl E, et al. Trends in smoking behaviour between 1985 and 2000 in nine European countries by education. J Epidemiol Community Heal. 2005 May 1;59(5):395-401.

42. Peter R, Siegrist J, Stork J, Mann H, Labrot B. [Cigarette smoking and psychosocial work stress in middle-management employees]. Soz Praventivmed. 1991;36(6):315-21.

43. Albertsen K, Borg V, Oldenburg B. A systematic review of the impact of work environment on smoking cessation, relapse and amount smoked. [Review] [50 refs].Preventive Medicine. 2006. p. 291-305.

44. Radi S, Ostry A, LaMontagne AD. Job stress and other working conditions: Relationships with smoking behaviors in a representative sample of working

Australians. Am J Ind Med. 2007 Aug;50(8):584-96.

45. Reward Deficiency Syndrome on JSTOR.

46. Chen M-J, Cunradi C. Job stress, burnout and substance use among urban transit operators: The potential mediating role of coping behaviour. Work Stress. Taylor & Francis Group ; 2008 Oct;22(4):327-40.

47. Jenkins CD, Zyzanski SJ, Rosenman RH. Biological, psychological, and social characteristics of men with different smoking habits. Health Serv Rep. Association of Schools of Public Health; 1973 Nov;88(9):834-43.

48. Shekelle RB, Schoenberger JA, Stamler J. Correlates of the JAS Type A behavior pattern score. J Chronic Dis. 1976 Jun;29(6):381-94.

49. Hiscock R, Dobbie F, Bauld L. Smoking Cessation and Socioeconomic Status: An Update of Existing Evidence from a National Evaluation of English Stop Smoking Services. Biomed Res Int. 2015;2015:274056.

50. Ota A, Masue T YN et al. Psychosocial job characteristics and smoking cessation: A prospective cohort study using the Demand;Control;Support and Effort;Reward Imbalance job stress models. Nicotine Tob Res. 2010;123:287-93.

51. Albertsen K, Hannerz H, Borg V, Burr H. Work environment and smoking cessation over a five-year period. Scand J Public Health. 2004 May;32(3):164-71.

APPENDICES

Observation sheet

SHEET N° :

Age

Years

Marital status: Single □ Married □ Divorced □ Widowed □ **Level of education:** Primary □ Secondary □Bac □ University □ **Profession:** **Length of service** years

Type of work: manual work □ office work □ field work □

Working hours: morning □ afternoon □ night □

Number of hours worked per week:

Breaks during work: no □ yes □

Habits :

Smoking: no □ yes □ Age at onset years

Still smoking □ Has stopped smoking □ In the process of cutting down □

Years of smoking:Number of cigarettes/day:Quantity PA

Type of tobacco: cigarette □ neffa □ hookah □

Do you smoke in the workplace? yes □ no □

If yes, when? during breaks □ outside breaks □

Are you aware of the health risks associated with smoking? yes □ no □

Have you been educated about smoking cessation in the last year? yes □ no□

Have you tried to stop smoking: no □ yes □ number of attempts:**Alcohol:** no □ yes □ Quantity:

Coffee: no □ yes □ number of coffees/day:

Medical history :

Cardiovascular diseases :

Hypertension □ Ischemic heart disease □ MI arteritis □ Other

Respiratory diseases :

COPD □Asthma □ DDB □ Chronic bronchitis □ Pneumonia □

Others

Cancer diseases :

KBP □ bladder □VADS □ Others:

Other antecedents:

Length of time off work for medical reasons over the last 12 months:

From which nature

ASSESSMENT OF CHEMICAL DEPENDENCE ON NICOTINE: FAGERSTRÖM QUESTIONNAIRE

How soon after waking up do you smoke your first cigarette?	Within the first 5 minutes	3
	Between 6 and 30 minutes	2
	Between 31 and 60 minutes	1
	After 60 minutes	0
Do you find it difficult to refrain from smoking in places where it is prohibited?	Yes	1
	No	0
Which cigarette would you find hardest to give up during the day?	First thing in the morning	1
	Any other	0
How many cigarettes do you smoke a day on average?	10 or less	0
	11 à 20	1
	21 à 30	2
	31 or more	3
Do you smoke more in the morning than in the afternoon?	Yes	1
	No	0
Do you smoke when you're ill, to the point of having to stay in bed most of the day?	Yes	1
	No	0
Total		

Dear Sir/Madam

Largue and Légeron test

Assessment of motivation

This questionnaire is designed to assess your motivation to stop smoking tobacco. Please fill it in, ticking one answer per line.

1- Do you think that in 6 months :

- You'll still smoke just as much	0
- You will have reduced your cigarette consumption slightly	2
- You will have significantly reduced your cigarette consumption	4
- You will have stopped smoking	8

2 - Do you currently want to stop smoking?

- Not at all	0
- A little	1
- Many	2
- Enormously	3

3 - Do you think that in 4 weeks :

- You'll still smoke just as much	0
- You will have reduced your cigarette consumption slightly	2
- You will have significantly reduced your cigarette consumption	4
- You will have stopped smoking	8

4 - Are you ever unhappy about smoking?

- never	0
- S ometimes	1
- Often	2
- always	3

Interpretation

< **6** insufficient motivation

7 to 13 average motivation

>**13** good motivation

French version of the Effort-Reward Imbalance questionnaire - 2004

For any use, please quote these two references:

Niedhammer I, Siegrist J, Landre MF, Goldberg M, Leclerc A. Etude des qualités psychométriques de la version française du modèle du Déséquilibre Efforts/Récompenses. Revue d'Epidémiologie et de Santé Publique 2000;48:419-437

Siegrist J, Starke D, Chandola T, Godin I, Marmot M, Niedhammer I, Peter R. The measurement of effort-reward imbalance at work: European comparisons. Social Science and Medicine 2004;58:1483-1499

1 I'm constantly pressed for time because of a heavy workload

Disagree倰$_1$ Agree, and I'm not disturbed at all............. 倰$_2$

Okay, and I'm a little confused .... 倰$_3$

Okay, and I'm confused .... 倰$_4$

Okay, and I'm very confused .... 倰$_5$

2 I am frequently interrupted and disturbed in the course of my work

Disagree倰$_1$ Agree, and I'm not disturbed at all............. 倰$_2$

Okay, and I'm a little confused .... 倰$_3$

Okay, and I'm confused .... 倰$_4$

Okay, and I'm very confused .... 倰$_5$

3 I have a lot of responsibility at work

No agreement .... 倰$_1$

Okay, and I'm not confused at all................................ 倰$_2$

Okay, and I'm a little confused .... 倰$_3$

Okay, and I'm confused .... 倰$_4$

Okay, and I'm very confused .... 倰$_5$

4 I'm often forced to work overtime

Disagree倰$_1$ Agree, and I'm not disturbed at all............. 倰$_2$

Okay, and I'm a little confused .... 倰$_3$

Okay, and I'm confused .... 倰$_4$

Okay, and I'm very confused .... 倰$_5$

5 My job requires physical effort

No agreement .... 倭₁

Okay, and I'm not confused at all .... 倭₂

Okay, and I'm a little confused .... 倭₃

Okay, and I'm confused .... 倭₄

Okay, and I'm very confused .... 倭₅

6 Over the last few years, my work has become increasingly demanding.

Disagree 倭₁ Agree, and I'm not disturbed at all .... 倭₂

Okay, and I'm a little confused .... 倭₃

Okay, and I'm confused .... 倭₄

Okay, and I'm very confused .... 倭₅

7 I get the respect I deserve from my superiors

Agreed .... 倭₁

Disagree, and I'm not at all disturbed .... **倭₂**

Disagree, and I'm a little disturbed .... 倭₃

I disagree, and I'm disturbed .... 倭₄

I disagree, and I'm very disturbed .... 倭₅

8 I get the respect I deserve from my colleagues

Agreed .... 倭₁

Disagree, and I'm not at all disturbed .... **倭₂**

Disagree, and I'm a little disturbed .... 倭₃

I disagree, and I'm disturbed .... 倭₄

I disagree, and I'm very disturbed .... 倭₅

9 At work, I receive satisfactory support in difficult situations

I agree 倭1

Disagree, and I'm not at all disturbed **倭2**

Disagree, and I'm a little disturbed. 倭3

I disagree, and I'm disturbed 倭4

I disagree, and I'm very disturbed 倭5

10 I'm treated unfairly at work

No agreement 倭1

Okay, and I'm not confused at all 倭2

Okay, and I'm a little confused 倭3

Okay, and I'm confused 倭4

Okay, and I'm very confused 倭5

11 I am experiencing or expecting an undesirable change in my life. work situation

No agreement 倭1

Okay, and I'm not confused at all 倭2

Okay, and I'm a little confused 倭3

Okay, and I'm confused 倭4

Okay, and I'm very confused 倭5

12 My prospects of promotion are poor

No agreement 倭1

Okay, and I'm not confused at all 倭2

Okay, and I'm a little confused 倭3

Okay, and I'm confused 倭4

Okay, and I'm very confused 倭5

13 My job security is under threat

No agreement 倭1

Okay, and I'm not confused at all....................................倭2

Okay, and I'm a little confused 倭3

Okay, and I'm confused 倭4

Okay, and I'm very confused 倭5

14 My current job corresponds well to my training

Agreed...倭1

Disagree, and I'm not at all disturbed 倭2

Disagree, and I'm a little disturbed.................................倭3

I disagree, and I'm disturbed...倭4

I disagree, and I'm very disturbed 倭5

15 Given all my efforts, I receive the respect and esteem I deserve for my work

Agreed...倭1

Disagree, and I'm not at all disturbed 倭2

Disagree, and I'm a little disturbed.................................倭3

I disagree, and I'm disturbed...倭4

I disagree, and I'm very disturbed 倭5

16 Given all my efforts, my prospects for promotion are good.

Agreed	倭1
I don't agree, and I'm not at all perturbed...	倭2
I disagree, and I'm a bit confused .. ..,	倭3
I disagree, and I'm disturbed	倭4
I disagree, and I'm very disturbed	倭5
17 Given all my efforts, my salary is satisfactory Agreed	倭1
I don't agree, and I'm not at all perturbed...	倭2
I disagree, and I'm a bit confused	倭3
I disagree, and I'm disturbed	倭4
I disagree, and I'm very disturbed	倭5

18At work, I often find myself

I totally disagree

No agreement

Agreed   Absolutely

Agreed

pressed for time...........................倭1倭2倭3倭4

19I'm starting to think about problems at

work as soon as I get up in the morning............倭1倭2倭3倭4

20When I get h o m e, it's easy for me to relax and forget about my work.

everything about my job..............倭1倭2倭3倭4

21Those close to me say I sacrifice too much

for my work..................................倭1倭2倭3倭4

22Work is still on my mind

when I go to bed.................................倭1倭2倭3倭4

23When I put off something that I should be doing on t h e day, I have a

hard time.

trouble sleeping at night..............................倭1倭2倭3倭4

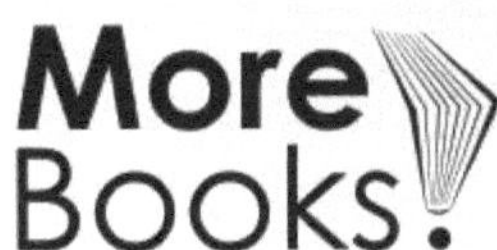

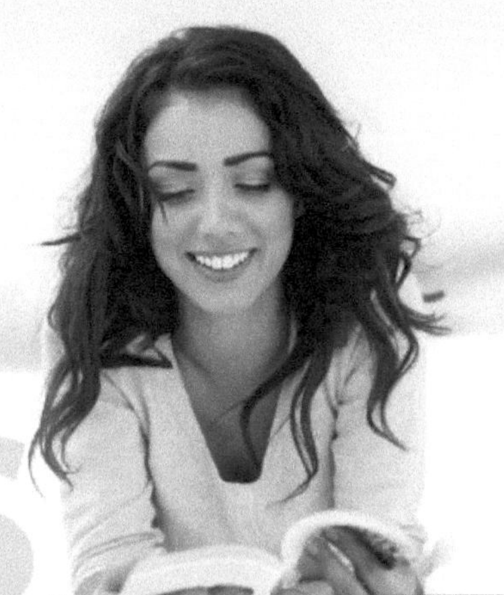

yes

I want morebooks!

Buy your books fast and straightforward online - at one of world's fastest growing online book stores! Environmentally sound due to Print-on-Demand technologies.

Buy your books online at
www.morebooks.shop

Kaufen Sie Ihre Bücher schnell und unkompliziert online – auf einer der am schnellsten wachsenden Buchhandelsplattformen weltweit! Dank Print-On-Demand umwelt- und ressourcenschonend produziert.

Bücher schneller online kaufen
www.morebooks.shop

info@omniscriptum.com
www.omniscriptum.com

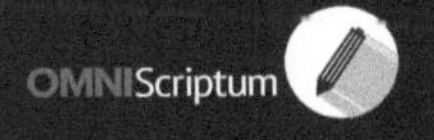

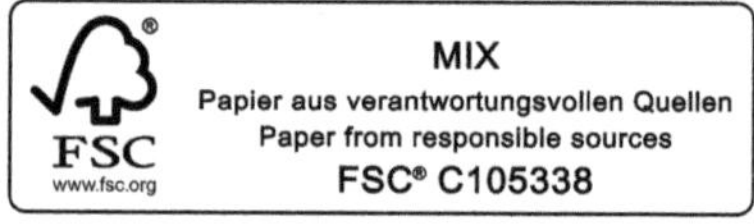

Printed by Books on Demand GmbH, Norderstedt / Germany